Pocket Calorie Guide
to Famous Foods

JANE COLIN'S

Pocket Calorie Guide to Famous Foods

London 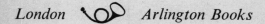 Arlington Books

POCKET CALORIE GUIDE TO
FAMOUS FOODS

*first published November 1972 by
Arlington Books (Publishers) Ltd.,
38 Bury Street, St James's,
London, S.W.1.*

*second impression July 1973
third impression April 1974*

© *Jane Colin* 1972

*Made and printed in England by
Wells KPL Swindon Press,
Swindon, Wiltshire.*

ISBN 85140 196 1

Contents

The Background to Slimming

Obesity is one of the diseases of affluence. Social and economic pressures tempt us to consume more all the time. As we eat more and walk less we become fatter, lazier and less healthy and the result is a vicious circle.

Not everyone who overeats is overweight. Some people don't put on weight whatever they eat, but most of us do put on weight, even if only very gradually, if the energy value of the food we eat is greater than the energy we use up in our daily life. This energy is measured in calories. It has been calculated that an excess of 20 calories a day—less than a teaspoon of sugar—could mean a gain of two pounds in body weight in a year.

The energy value of food, of course, is not the only consideration. Carbohydrate and fat are primarily energy-supplying foods but for a balanced diet we need protein to keep the body in good repair, as well as vitamins, minerals and so on. It is always important to see that you get a wide variety of foods but particularly so when you are on a low-calorie diet. Generally it is safest to cut down on carbohydrate foods first, then fats. You may be able to keep your protein consumption much the same as it usually is. Most people lose quite a lot at the beginning of a diet so it is best to keep something in reserve so that you can cut down further when your weight loss begins to slow up. Starvation dieting is unwise except for the odd day and there is some evidence that it is not the most effective way to lose weight quickly. It is best to begin around 1200 or even 1500 calories a day and then cut down gradually but never below 700. Remember that even 100 calories a day less could take off a pound in a month and a slow and steady weight loss is easier to maintain.

Although the selection of "Famous Foods" has been as wide as possible, there are obviously many well known foods which could not be included without making the book too big to be useful. If you can't find a particular brand, you should be able to find something else comparable which will give you a good idea of the calorie value of the brand you prefer.

This book is primarily designed to help people who are trying to lose weight by enabling them to choose amongst a much wider variety of foods than is usually included on the standard slimming diet. But anyone who has had to diet would agree that it is far better not to put on weight in the first place. One of the best ways of doing this is to have a good knowledge of the calorie value of foods so that you can keep a proper balance between your energy expenditure and energy intake. So this book is also intended for people who are not actually trying to get thinner but feel they might easily become overweight if they are not fairly careful. For this reason, I have included some foods which would be best avoided by anyone on a real slimming diet.

As far as possible I have tried to give the quantities in a standard form so that it is fairly easy to compare one food with another, and to calculate how many calories there are in your own helpings. For people who have no means of weighing, there is usually some indication of the size of helping either in spoonfuls or cups or as a proportion of the can or packet in which it is sold.* Tablespoons and so on are not an accurate way of measuring but it is a lot better to measure this way than not to measure at all. In fact, many people find that simply calculating the calories and keeping a record is enough to help them to lose weight without needing to go on a strict diet.

You may already have a copy of Jane Colin's *Pocket Calorie Guide to Safe Slimming*, published in 1965. This covers the general background to slimming in more detail and gives the calorie values of basic foods in their natural state. It is possible to use *The Pocket Calorie Guide to Famous Foods* on its own but the two do complement each other and I have indicated when fuller information on certain points is available in *The Pocket Calorie Guide to Safe Slimming*.

* *Cans and packets should always be marked with the weight or volume of their contents which will help you to check.*

WHAT YOU SHOULD WEIGH

The following table gives you the *average* weight for your height. But don't blindly make this your goal. Individual weights vary according to bone structure and your own ideal weight may be as much as half a stone different.

First of all, weigh yourself and compare your weight with the chart. Then judge your frame type. You probably have a good idea, anyway, but you can check this by wrist measurements. For a man—up to $6\frac{1}{2}''$ indicates a small frame, up to $7''$ a medium frame and above $7''$ a large frame. For a woman, $5\frac{1}{2}''$ indicates a small frame, $6''$ a medium frame and over $6\frac{1}{2}''$ a large frame.

If you are large-framed and heavy boned you may look too thin at the average weight. If you are small-framed and light-boned, you may still look too fat at the average weight. Provided that you are within half a stone of the average weight, you are quite safe, medically speaking. After that it is up to you to find out the weight at which you feel your best and look your best. Then your aim should be to get there and *stay there!*

AVERAGE WEIGHTS TABLE

(These include light clothing, but no shoes. If you weigh unclothed, deduct 3lbs from the weight shown here).

MEN			WOMEN	
Height Ft. Ins.	Weight St. lbs.		Height Ft. Ins.	Weight St. lbs.
5 0	9 0		4 8	8 0
5 1	9 2		4 9	8 2
5 2	9 4		4 10	8 4
5 3	9 7		4 11	8 6
5 4	9 10		5 0	8 8
5 5	10 0		5 1	8 10
5 6	10 4		5 2	8 12
5 7	10 8		5 3	9 1
5 8	10 12		5 4	9 5
5 9	11 2		5 5	9 8
5 10	11 7		5 6	9 12
5 11	11 12		5 7	10 2
6 0	12 4		5 8	10 6
6 1	12 10		5 9	10 10
6 2	13 2		5 10	11 0
6 3	13 8		5 11	11 3
6 4	14 0		6 0	11 7

Cereal Products

In affluent societies, consumption of cereals tends to go down and more luxurious foods such as meat, fats and sugar are chosen instead. This is certainly more expensive and may not always be an advantage to health. Cereals are often identified with carbohydrates but in fact they are the main source of protein in many of the poorer countries and they are also important for a number of vitamins and minerals. It is unwise to cut them out completely even on a low calorie diet but they do need to be watched. They are not specially high in calories in themselves but it is easy to eat them in large quantities and the total can become very high indeed when you add milk, butter, cream, jam, sugar and so on.

Food	Quantities	Calories
BREADS AND CRISPBREADS		
Allinson Starch-reduced		
rolls—white	1 roll	18
—brown	1 roll	21
100% wholewheat bread	1 oz slice	64
B.N. French Toasts	1 toast	30
Bread—average	1 oz (medium slice)	70
Energen Starch-reduced		
wheat crispbread	1 piece	26
rye crispbread	1 piece	25
cheese crispbread	1 piece	25
roll	1 roll	27
Granose Starch-reduced rolls	1 roll	21

Food	Quantities	Calories
Ry-King		
Slim light crispbread	1 piece	28
Brown Rye crispbread	1 piece	33
Wheat crispbread	1 piece	38
Ryvita	1 piece	28
Scanda Brod	1 piece	32
,, Crisp	1 piece	19
Breakfast Cereals		
Alpen Mixed Cereal	1 oz	105
Bird's Grape Nuts	1 oz	100
Energen Starch-reduced		
Wheat Flakes	1 oz	113
Force Wheat Flakes	1 oz	105
Fruti-Fort—Swiss Bircher-		
Muesli	1 oz	114
Granose Fruit Bran	1 oz	104
,, Sunnybisk	1 oz (approx. 2 biscuits)	106
Kellogg's All Bran	1 oz	88
,, Bran Buds	1 oz	95
,, Bran Flakes	1 oz	99
,, Coco Krispies	1 oz	105
,, Corn Flakes	1 oz	102
,, Frosties	1 oz	103
,, Puffa Puffa Rice	1 oz	119
,, Raisin Bran	1 oz	98
,, Rice Krispies	1 oz	101
,, Ricicles	1 oz	101
,, Special K	1 oz	102
,, Sugar Smacks	1 oz	105
Kollath Wheat Flakes	1 oz	100

Food	Quantities	Calories
Lyons Ready Brek	1 oz	106
Millotto	1 oz	120
Millett Flakes	1 oz	102
Quaker Puffed Wheat	1 oz	102
,, Quick Quaker Oats	1 oz (dry weight)	115
Shredded Wheat	1 biscuit	93
,, ,, Spoonsize	1 oz (16 biscuits)	116
Shreddies	1 oz	116
Weetabix	1 biscuit	60
	1 oz	100

Dairy Foods, Fats and Oils

Dairy Foods are very important nutritionally and should play quite a large part in any diet, whether or not you are trying to lose weight. Milk is an almost perfect food because it supplies most of the essential nutritional elements, apart from Vitamin C and iron, in good quantities and it is wise to see that you have at least half a pint a day. Cheese is a good source of protein and calcium and is nutritionally about as valuable as the best rump steak. Eggs at 80-90 calories each according to size are another good source of protein, vitamins and minerals and are, nevertheless, a comparatively low calorie food. Fats and oils, on the other hand, are very concentrated, high calorie foods. Because they are not bulky and are often consumed in a disguised form—for example fat used in frying or in ice-creams and cakes—they can add greatly to your total calorie consumption without your being aware of having eaten at all excessively. If you have a weight problem or are trying to lose weight, fats should be watched very carefully and strictly limited. They are a good source of energy and help to create a feeling of satisfaction after a meal because they stay longer in the stomach and they are an essential part of a normal diet, but even if you are not worried about weight large amounts of fat and fatty foods can be bad for both health and beauty.

Food	Quantities	Calories
MILKS		
Fresh, full cream milk—ave.	Half pint	190
Carnation Coffee Mate	$\frac{1}{4}$ oz powder	40
	Half pint reconstituted	162
Carnation Milk	$\frac{1}{4}$ pint undiluted	245
Fussells Skimmed Sweetened Milk	1 oz (1$\frac{1}{2}$ tablespns.)	78
Ideal Full Cream Evaporated Milk	$\frac{1}{4}$ pint undiluted	235
Marvel	$\frac{1}{4}$ oz powder (1 teaspoon)	25
	Half pint reconstituted	100
Nestle's Full Cream Sweetened Condensed Milk	1 oz (1$\frac{1}{2}$ tablespns.)	96
Nestle's Instant Skimmed Milk Powder	$\frac{1}{4}$ oz (1 teaspoon)	25
Regal Full Cream Evaporated Milk	$\frac{1}{4}$ pint undiluted	235
CREAMS		
Nestle's Cream	1 oz (1$\frac{1}{2}$ tablespns.)	68
St. Ivel Double Cream	,, ,,	128
,, ,, Devon Cream	,, ,,	128
YOGURTS		
Alpine Fruit Yoghurt— average for all flavours	5 oz carton	90
Eden Vale Natural Yogurt	5 oz carton	77
Fat Free Yogurt	5 oz carton	69
Banana, Coffee, Lemon, Raspberry, Strawberry–all	5 oz carton	119

Food	Quantities	Calories
Chocolate, Choc-Lemon, Choc-Strawberry, Choc-Raspberry—all	5 oz carton	190
St. Ivel Natural Yogurt	,, ,,	90
,, ,, Super Fruit Yogurt	6 oz carton	180
Ski Yogurt	,, ,,	175
CHEESE		
Dairylea Cheese Spread	1 oz	78
,, Processed Cheese Portions	1 oz	78
Eden Vale Cottage Cheese	,,	30
Kraft Cheeze Whiz and other Kraft cheese spreads—all	1 oz	78
Kraft De-Luxe Slices	,,	98
St. Ivel Cottage Cheese	,,	32
Swiss Knight Cheese Spread	,,	78
,, ,, Processed Cheeses	1 oz	95
Velveeta Cheese Spread	,,	78
,, Processed Cheese portions	1 oz	87
FATS & COOKING OILS		
Butter—average	1 oz	220
Margarines		
Flora	1 oz	226
Soft Blue Band	,,	226
Stork	,,	226
Summer County	,,	226
Tomor	,,	226
Outline low fat spread	,,	108
Oils		
Mazola Corn Oil	1 fl. oz (1½ tbsps)	252
Olive Oil—average	,, ,,	252

Food	Quantities	Calories
Sun-O-Life Sunflower Seed Oil	1 fl. oz (1½ tbsps)	261
Trex Vegetable Oil	,, ,,	180
Twirl Vegetable Oil	,, ,,	180
Cooking Fats		
Cookeen	1 oz	262
Lard—average	,,	262
Spry	,,	262
Trex	,,	260
White Cap	,,	262

Soups

The nutritional value of soups varies so widely according to what they are made with that it is impossible to generalise. A hot soup gives a feeling of comfort and relaxation and so aids digestion as well as making sandwiches or a cold meal very much more attractive. For people trying to lose weight or keep it down, hot, thin soup is low in calories and, by taking the edge off your appetite, will help to reduce the amount of food you want to eat during the rest of the meal and still leave you feeling satisfied.

Food	Quantities		Calories
SOUPS AND STOCK CUBES			
Batchelors			
Asparagus	¼ pint (1½ ladles)		52
Barbecue Beef and Tomato	,,	,,	40
Chicken Noodle	,,	,,	30
Country Chicken and Leek	,,	,,	48
Garden Vegetable	,,	,,	20
Golden Vegetable	,,	,,	51
Harvest Vegetable	,,	,,	65
Minestrone	,,	,,	38
Mushroom	,,	,,	48
Oxtail	,,	,,	40
Savoury Beef and Onion	,,	,,	40
Scotch Broth	,,	,,	50
Thick Chicken	,,	,	68
Thick Devon Onion	,,	,,	48
Thick Farmhouse Vegetable	¼ pint (1½ ladles)		38

Food	Quantities	Calories
Thick Lincoln Pea	¼ pint (1½ ladles)	68
Tomato	,, ,,	50
Traditional Vegetable and Beef	¼ pint (1½ ladles)	40
Crosse & Blackwell		
Beef	¼ pint (1½ ladles)	70
Consommé	,, ,,	30
Cottage Style Potato	,, ,,	95
Country Vegetable & Beef	,, ,,	55
Cream of Chicken	,, ,,	70
Cream of Chicken & Ham	,, ,,	100
Cream of Mushroom	,, ,,	70
Creamed Tomato	,, ,,	95
Cream of Vegetable	,, ,,	80
Farmhouse	,, ,,	80
Harvest Cream	,, ,,	85
Minestrone	,, ,,	90
Oxtail	,, ,,	70
Scotch Broth	,, ,,	80
Vegetable	,, ,,	70
Heinz		
Beef Broth	⅓ can (app. ¼ pint)	54
Beef Soup	,, ,,	66
Beef Steak and Kidney	,, ,,	60
Clear Chicken Broth	,, ,,	22
Country Broth	,, ,,	44
Consommé	,, ,,	28
Cream of Asparagus	,, ,,	84
Cream of Celery	,, ,,	67
Cream of Chicken	,, ,,	94
Cream of Mushroom	,, ,,	71
Cream of Tomato	,, ,,	101
Cream of Turkey	,, ,,	82
Golden Chicken and Leek	,, ,,	29

Food	Quantities		Calories
Kidney	⅓ can (app. ¼ pint)		57
Lentil	,,	,,	69
Minestrone	,,	,,	69
Mulligatawny	,,	,,	76
Oxtail	,,	,,	65
Pea and Ham	,,	,,	69
Scotch Broth	,,	,,	48
Scottish Vegetable	,,	,,	76
Spring Vegetable	,,	,,	52
Thick Chicken with Vegetables	⅓ can (app. ¼ pint)		64
Thick Vegetable and Beef Broth	⅓ can (app. ¼ pint)		84
Vegetable	,,	,,	52
Knorr			
Chicken	¼ pint (1½ ladles) as reconstituted		40
Chicken & Leek	,,	,,	34
Chicken & Vegetable	,,	,,	34
Country Vegetable	,,	,,	41
Florida Spring Vegetable	,,	,,	22
Leek	,,	,,	36
Minestrone	,,	,,	27
Mushroom	,,	,,	61
Oxtail	,,	,,	31
Super Chicken Noodle	,,	,,	33
Thick Asparagus	,,	,,	40
Thick Country Pea	,,	,,	58
Thick Tomato	,,	,,	62
Maggi			
Beef Stock Tablets	¼ pint (1½ ladles) as reconstituted		8
Chicken Noodle	,,	,,	34

Food	Quantities		Calories
Chicken Stock Tablets	¼ pint (1½ ladles) as reconstituted		9
Country Vegetable	,,	,,	36
Minestrone	,,	,,	45
Mushroom	,,	,,	35
Oxtail	,,	,,	41
Pea with Smoked Ham	,,	,,	40
Scotch Broth	,,	,,	42
Spring Vegetable	,,	,,	30
Thick Chicken	,,	,,	45
Thick Vegetable with Beef	,,	,,	34
Tomato	,,	,,	51
Tomato Vegetable	,,	,,	32
Oxo			
Golden Oxo Cube	1 cube		13
Red Oxo Cube	,,		13

Fish — Canned and Frozen

There is a limited range of canned fish and most of it varies very little in calorie content from the quantities given in the list of basic foods in *Jane Colin's Pocket Calorie Guide*. Fish is a valuable source of protein and has the advantage of being low in fat and therefore relatively low in calories. Even if you are following quite a strict slimming diet you can still have a good helping of fish but you must remember that frying, rich sauces and mayonnaises can soon transform a basically low calorie food into a very high calorie helping.

Food	Quantities	Calories
FISH		
Crosse & Blackwell Canned		
Herrings in Tomato Sauce	Half 7 oz can	157
John West Canned		
Crab	Half 6½ oz can	117
Kipper	Half 7 oz can	199
Salmon	Half 7½ oz can	146
Sardines	Half 4½ oz can	189
Shrimps	Half 4½ oz can	80
Tuna	Half 7½ oz can	255
Bird's Eye Frozen		
Buttered Kipper Fillets	Half 6 oz packet	150
Buttered Smoke Haddock	Half 7½ oz pack	110
Cod in Butter Sauce	1 individual packet	200
Cod in Cheese Sauce	,, ,,	180
Cod in Shrimp Flavour		
Sauce	1 individual packet	155

Food	Quantities	Calories
Cod Steaks in Breadcrumbs	1 steak	135
Crispy Cod Fries	Half 7 oz pack	160
Fish Cakes	1 fish cake	65
Fish Fingers	1 fish finger	55
Haddock Steaks in Breadcrumbs	1 steak	125
Findus Frozen		
Breaded Plaice	1 portion	96
Buttered Kipper Fillets	Half 6 oz pack	195
Buttered Smoked Haddock	Half 7½ oz pack	94
Cod Fillets	Half 13 oz pack	157
Cod Portions (Breaded)	1 portion	64
Cod Steaks (Unbreaded)	1 steak	69
Fish Cakes	1 cake	68
Fish Fingers	1 finger	49
Haddock Fillets	Half 13 oz pack	150
Haddock Portions (Breaded)	1 portion	62
Plaice Fillets	6 oz pack	144
Rainbow Trout	Half 12 oz pack	216
Ross Frozen		
Breaded Cod Steaks	1 steak	141
Breaded Hake Portions	1 steak	110
Cod in Batter	1 portion	226
Cod in Butter Sauce	6 oz pack	145
Fish Cakes	1 cake	68
Fish Fingers	1 finger	46
Salmon Fish Cakes	1 cake	84

Meat

Meat is one of our main sources of protein and other important nutritional elements, but cereals, nuts, beans and peas also contribute protein and other useful elements. Even if you could afford to live exclusively on best quality steaks you would be much wiser to choose a more varied diet. Overweight is rarely due to the kind of foods included in this section, unless you have a very large appetite, and they should not need to be cut down at all drastically for a slimming diet. Keep an eye on the total calories consumed and avoid foods that have a very high fat content.

Food	Quantities	Calories
MEATS, PIES AND READY MEALS		
Crosse & Blackwell		
Baked Beans	5 oz tin	140
Ham and Beef Roll	4 ozs	240
Ham and Chicken Roll	4 ozs	252
Spaghetti Rings in Tomato Sauce	7½ oz can	123
Snack Meals		
Beans and Hamburgers	5 ozs	170
Country Supper	,,	165
Noodles and Chicken Capri	,,	145
London Grill	,,	220
Spaghetti and Beef Roma	,,	165
Chef		
Beans and Bacon	Half 8 oz tin	140
Beans and Pork	,, ,, ,, ,,	144

Food	Quantities	Calories
Duo-Can (Harveys)		
Beef Curry	1 small tin	389
Chicken Curry	„ „ „	378
Fray Bentos		
Braised Steak in gravy	5 ozs	375
Corned Beef	3 ozs	215
Mild Curried Beef	5 ozs	235
Mild Curried Chicken	5 ozs	235
Minced Steak pie filling	5 ozs	400
Ox tongue	3 ozs	265
Savoury minced steak with onion	5 ozs	400
Steak and kidney pie	5 ozs	435
Steak and kidney pudding	5 ozs	375
Steak and kidney pie filling	5 ozs	400
Steak and Mushroom pie filling	5 ozs	300
Steak and onion pie filling	5 ozs	400
Granose		
Nutmeat Brawn	4 oz serving	148
Nutmeat	4 oz serving	204
Nuttolene	3 oz serving	282
Rissol-Nut	1 oz	129
Saviand	4 oz serving	204
C. & T. Harris		
Pies		
Cornish Pasty	1 individual	304
Minced Beef	¼ of family size pie	353
Pork	1 mini size	289
	1 individual	514
Steak & Kidney	„ „	539
Sausages		
Standard Pork	1 sausage	207
	1 chipolata	103

Food	Quantities	Calories
Standard Pork & Beef	1 sausage	169
	1 chipolata	85
Crown Brand Pork	1 sausage	233
Savoury Specialities		
Black Pudding	2 ozs	174
Faggots	2 ozs	219
Liver & Bacon Croquettes	1 croquette	118
Liver Sausage	2 ozs	173
Polony	2 ozs	190
Canned Products		
Beef Mince with Onions and Gravy	half 15½ oz can	404
4 Beef burgers with Onions and Gravy	half 15½ oz can	263
Chunky Steak & Gravy	,, ,, ,,	344
High Tea (beans & baconburgers)	half 8 oz can	192
Ox Tongue—butt	¼ of 16 oz can	336
,, ,, —tip	half 8 oz can	160
Pork Brawn	half 7½ oz can	328
Savoury Minced Steak with Gravy	7 oz can	419
Savoury Minced Steak with Gravy	5 oz can	299
Steak & Kidney Pie	half 15½ oz can	388
Sweetcure Ham	¼ of 16 oz can	155
Wiltshire Pork Sausage	1 sausage	121
Heinz		
Erin		
Beef Curry with Rice	1 serving can	407
Chicken Bombay with Rice	1 serving can	357
Beef Casserole with Potato Dumplings	1 serving can	353

Food	Quantities	Calories
Savoury Beef in Potato Nests	1 serving can	314
Chicken Casserole	,, ,,	332
Beef Continental	,, ,,	311
Ready Meals		
Beef & Vegetable Curry	8 oz can	231
Lamb & Vegetable Curry	,, ,,	265
Beans		
Baked Beans	half 7¾ oz can	95
Beans & Baconburgers	half 7½ oz can	106
Beans and Frankfurters	,, ,, ,, ,,	135
Beans & Minced Beef	,, ,, ,, ,,	109
Beans & Sausages	half 7¾ oz can	141
Curried Beans	,, ,, ,, ,,	112
Pasta varieties		
Macaroni with Cheese Sauce	half 7¼ oz can	119
Ravioli	,, ,, ,, ,,	96
Spaghetti Bolognese	,, ,, ,, ,,	68
Spaghetti Hoops with Beef Sauce	half 7¼ oz can	53
Spaghetti Hoops with Tomato Sauce	half 7½ oz can	54
Spaghetti with Tomato & Cheese Sauce	half 7½ oz can	69
Plumrose		
Bacon Grill	4 ozs	344
Chopped Ham with Pork	,,	340
Cocktail Sausages	1 sausage	17
Cooked Boneless Ham	4 ozs	136
Frankfurter Sausages	1 sausage	50
Hot Dog Sausages	1 sausage	45
Luncheon Meat	4 ozs	386
Party Sausages	1 sausage	18
Pork Luncheon Meat	4 ozs	386

Food	Quantities	Calories
Smedley's Sausage Rolls	1 oz	85
Vesta Complete Meals		
Beef Curry	8 oz portion	280
Chicken Curry	,, ,,	214
Chicken Supreme	,, ,,	237
Chow Mein	,, ,,	246
Paella	,, ,,	180
Prawn Curry	,, ,,	206
Spaghetti Bolognese	7 oz portion	200
Vegetable Curry	8 oz portion	220
T. Wall & Sons		
Pies		
Grosvenor (with eggs)	One 5 oz slice	545
Raised	,, ,, ,,	600
Small pork pie	1 pie	590
Small steak and kidney	,,	630
Sausages		
Beef or meat	1 sausage	150
Pork	,,	216
Canned Products		
Pork luncheon meat	half 7 oz can	332
Stewed steak with gravy	half 15 oz can	330
FROZEN MEATS, PIES AND		
READY MEALS		
Bird's Eye		
Beefburgers	1 beefburger	160
Beefburgers with cheese	1 ,,	160
Chicken pie	1 individual	400
Chicken & Ham pie	1 ,,	400
Chicken & Mushroom		
Casserole	1 individual pack	135

Food	Quantities	Calories
Chicken Rissoles	1 rissole	145
Gravy & Roast Pork with stuffing	One 3¾ oz pack	120
Meat and Potato pie	1 individual	350
Minced Beef & Onion pie	1 ,,	350
Porkburgers	1 porkburger	140
Pork Rissoles	1 rissole	155
Roast Beef Dinner	1 individual pack	390
Roast Chicken Dinner	1 individual pack	300
Roast Chicken & Sausage with Stuffing & Gravy	One 4¾ oz pack	120
Sausage Rolls	1 roll	150
Savoury Rissoles	1 rissole	160
Scotch Rissoles	1 ,,	160
Shepherds Pie	1 individual tray	225
Sliced Roast Beef in Gravy	One 4 oz pack	120
Steak & Kidney Pie	1 individual	400
Steaklets	1 steaklet	190
Turkey Pie	1 individual	350
Findus		
Beefburgers	1 beefburger	140
Faggots in Gravy	1 faggot with gravy	147
Shepherds Pie	One 8 oz pack	248
Sliced Braised Beef	1 portion (4½ ozs)	140
Ross		
Beef burgers	1 beefburger	184
Beef Casserole	half 8 oz pack	86
Chicken à la King		88
Chicken Pie	One 5 oz pie	557
Cornish Pasties	1 pasty	294
Family Beef Steak Pie	Quarter of 16 oz pack	357

Food	Quantities	Calories
Minced Steak Pie	One 5 oz pie	560
Pork Sausages	1 sausage	88
Sausage Rolls	1 roll	121
Sliced Roast Beef in Gravy	One 4 oz pack	93
Steaklets	1 steaklet	210

Note.—The calorie values given refer to the foods as purchased and do not make any allowance for fat or other ingredients added when the product is cooked.

Vegetables

Most frozen and canned vegetables have the same calorie values as the fresh products which are covered in more detail in *Jane Colin's Pocket Calorie Guide*. However the calorie content, with a few exceptions, is so low that it need not be of much concern. Vegetables are a prime source of Vitamin C and, as this is a vitamin we don't store in the body, they should be eaten in good quantities every day. If you are on a fairly strict slimming diet, vegetables are useful for adding variety and bulk. As always with low calorie foods, it is easy to add fats and sauces and end up with a high calorie count—for example, boiled onions are 4 calories to the ounce but fried onions 101 calories to the ounce.

Food	Quantities	Calories
Baked Beans—see Meats and Ready Meals section		
Findus Frozen		
Asparagus	Half 8 oz pack	28
Broad Beans	Half 8 oz pack	144
Broccoli	Third 9 oz pack	27
Brussels Sprouts	4 oz pack	44
Corn on the Cob	1 cob	195
Crinkle Cut Chips	Half 6 oz pack	135
Haricots Verts	Half 8 oz pack	33
Mixed Vegetables	,, ,,	68
Peas (including Petits Pois)	4 oz pack	80
Ratatouille	Half 14 oz pack	94

Food	Quantities	Calories
Sliced Green Beans	4 oz pack	33
Spinach (whole leaf)	Half 8 oz pack	33
Sweet Corn	Half 6 oz pack	78
Heinz Canned		
Potato Salad	Half 7½ oz can	202
Vegetable Salad	,, ,,	145
Smedleys Canned		
Beetroot	5 ozs	40
Broad Beans	,,	50
Butter Beans	,,	105
Carrots	,,	30
Celery Hearts	,,	6
Garden Peas	,,	85
Green Beans	,,	16
Mixed Vegetables	,,	50
New Potatoes	,,	75
Processed Peas	,,	80
Red Kidney Beans	,,	100
Spinach	,,	16

Fruit

Fruit is a useful source of Vitamin C and makes an important contribution to the general diet. It is particularly valuable to anyone on a slimming diet because it is low in calories and yet helps to satisfy the desire for something sweet. You can find details about the calorie values of individual fresh fruits in *Jane Colin's Pocket Calorie Guide* to basic foods. In most cases, frozen fruit can be regarded as equivalent to fresh fruit. Canned fruit differs mainly because of the sugar content in the syrup—the short list given here can be taken as representative of most brands.

Food	*Quantities*	*Calories*
FRUIT		
(Diabetic products are sweetened with products which are more suitable than ordinary sugar for diabetics but are not necessarily lower in calories)		
Frank Cooper Diabetic Products		
Apricots	4 oz portion	56
Fruit Salad	,, ,,	58
Peaches	,, ,,	58
Pears	,, ,,	56
Pineapple	,, ,,	62
John West		
Apricot halves	$\frac{1}{3}$ of 15$\frac{1}{2}$ oz can	155
Fruit Cocktail	. ,, ,,	139
Fruit salad	,, ,,	139

Food	Quantities		Calories
Mandarin oranges	⅓ of 11 oz can		66
Peach halves	⅓ of 15½ oz can		129
Peach slices	,,	,,	129
Pear halves	,,	,,	114
Pineapple	,,	,,	117
Libby's			
Apricots	3 heaped tbsps. (5 ozs approx.)		120
Cling Peaches	,,	,,	110
Fruit Cocktail	,,	,,	105
Grapefruit Segments	,,	,,	100
Pears	,,	,,	105
Pineapple	,,	,,	100
Smedley's			
Apple Puree	,,	,,	100
Apricots	,,	,,	116
Blackberries	,,	,,	119
Blackcurrants	,,	,,	119
Fruit Cocktail	,,	,,	100
Fruit Salad	,,	,,	100
Gooseberries	,,	,,	109
Loganberries	,,	,,	113
Peaches	,,	,,	100
Pears	,,	,,	97
Plums	,,	,,	110
Prunes	,,	,,	132
Raspberries	,,	,,	117
Rhubarb	,,	,,	106
Strawberries	,,	,,	113

Puddings

Puddings add enormously to the variety of meals. They can also add enormously to your weight if you are not careful. The important thing is to consider the overall content of the meal. If you want to have a good hearty steamed pudding then choose fish or an omelette or something else fairly low in calories for your first course. If you are trying to lose weight, fresh fruit is a sensible choice for pudding but you can make a change with tinned fruit and a little cream or ice cream and some of the lighter whips and mousses could probably be fitted in to your calorie allowance.

Food	Quantities	Calories
Cadbury Schweppes Appletree Desserts		
—average for all flavours	5 ozs (approx. one third packet made up)	90
Bird's		
Angel Delight—Banana, Coffee, Raspberry, Strawberry	¼ 2 oz pack made up	140
Angel Delight		
Butterscotch	¼ 2 oz pack made up	137
Chocolate	¼ 3 oz pack made up	154
Orange, Lemon, Lime	¼ 2 oz pack made up	137
Custard Powder	½ oz powder (1 tablespoon)	50

Food	Quantities	Calories
	$\frac{1}{4}$ pint made up	175
Dream Topping	1 packet (1 oz)	320
	1 heaped tbspn. made up	30
Instant Whip—Banana, Orange, Raspberry, Strawberry, Vanilla	$\frac{1}{4}$ $3\frac{1}{4}$ oz pack made up	187
Instant Whip— Butterscotch, Lemon	$\frac{1}{4}$ 3 oz pack made up	177
Chocolate	$\frac{1}{4}$ 3 oz pack made up	185
Lemon Pie Filling	1 $2\frac{3}{4}$ oz packet (egg and pastry must be added for total)	380
Bird's Eye Frozen		
Chocolate Cream Sponge	One eighth of cake	105
Dairy Cream Sponge	,, ,, ,, ,,	100
Eclairs	One eclair	135
Puff Pastry	1 oz as purchased	115
Short Crust Pastry	,, ,, ,, ,,	130
Brown & Polson Flavoured Blancmange—average for all	4 oz portion made up	124
Chivers		
Chocolate Jelly-Cream	$\frac{1}{4}$ pint made up	152
Jelly-Creams except chocolate	$\frac{1}{4}$ pint made up	159
Table jellies	,, ,, ,, ,,	100
Crosse & Blackwell		
Chocolate Pudding	$\frac{1}{3}$ of $10\frac{1}{2}$ oz can	297
Date Pudding	,, ,, ,, ,,	290
Golden Pudding	,, ,, ,, ,,	290

Food	Quantities	Calories
Marmalade Pudding	⅓ of 10½ oz can	294
Mixed Fruit Pudding	,, ,, ,, ,,	283
Sultana Pudding	,, ,, ,, ,,	294
Cow & Gate Creamed Rice	6 oz can	180
Eden Vale Fruit Fool		
Blackcurrant	1 carton	68
Raspberry	,,	70
Strawberry	,,	76
Findus Frozen Mousses		
Chocolate	5 ozs	220
Lemon	,,	230
Strawberry	,,	210
Heinz		
Chocolate Pudding	⅓ of 10½ oz can	290
Ginger Pudding	,, ,, ,, ,,	313
Golden Honey Pudding	,, ,, ,, ,,	305
Mixed Fruit	,, ,, ,, ,,	306
Raspberry	,, ,, ,, ,,	278
Sultana	,, ,, ,, ,,	325
Treacle	,, ,, ,, ,,	330
Lyons Pudding Mixes		
Batter Mix	1 oz made up but uncooked	44
Sponge pudding	,, ,, ,,	97
Unsweetened pudding	,, ,, ,,	101
Sweetened pudding	,, ,, ,,	97
Short pastry mix	,, ,, ,,	108
Morton Pie Fillings		
Apple & Blackberry	Fifth of 14 oz can	77
Apple	,, ,, ,, ,,	75
Apricot	,, ,, ,, ,,	62
Blackcurrant	,, ,, ,, ,,	82
Cherry	,, ,, ,, ,,	80

Food	Quantities	Calories
Gooseberry	Fifth of 14 oz can	64
Nabisco Simply Sweet Desserts		
Apple Sponge	4 ozs made up	168
Apple & Blackberry Sponge	4 ozs made up	168
Apple & Raspberry Crumble	4 ozs made up	196
Lemon Meringue Crunch	3 ozs made up	216
Ross Frozen		
Apple Pie	¼ 14 oz pack	294
Blackcurrant Mousse	3½ oz indiv. pack	92
Butterscotch Mousse	,, ,, ,,	95
Chocolate Ripple Mousse	,, ,, ,,	97
Creme Caramel	4 oz indiv. pack	167
Custard Pie	¼ 14 oz pack	255
Dairy Cream Sponge	¼ 8 oz pack	202
Dairy Cream Trifle	3¾ oz indiv. pack	212
Raspberry Ripple Mousse	3½ oz indiv. pack	91
Raspberry and Vanilla Mousse	3½ oz indiv. pack	87
Strawberry Mousse	,, ,, ,,	89
Suisse Delice	⅓ 6½ oz pack	145
Rowntree's Table Jellies Royal	¼ pint made up	100
Chiffon	2¾ oz packet not made up	268
	Eggs added—each	90
Pie Fillings	2¾ oz packet not made up	268
	Eggs added—each	90
	Short pastry average unckd 1 oz	132

Food	Quantities	Calories
Whisk-it	3½ oz packet	362
	¼ pint made up with milk	190
St. Ivel Fresh Cream Desserts		
Chocolate	4½ oz carton	265
Coffee	,, ,,	252
Fruit	,, ,,	220
Viota		
Economix Crumble	Sixth of a packet made up without fruit	182
Economix Pastry	Sixth of a packet made up, no filling	185
Honeycomb Mould		
standard	Sixth of a packet made up	135
chocolate	Sixth of a packet made up	142
raspberry	Sixth of a packet made up	138
Whip		
chocolate	Sixth of a packet made up	123
raspberry	Sixth of a packet made up	119
strawberry	Sixth of a packet made up	119
vanilla	Sixth of a packet made up	119
Walls Individual Desserts		
Blackberry and Apple	1 individual	103
Chocolate Fool	,,	118

Food	Quantities	Calories
Chocolate Mousse	1 individual	104
Chocolate & Pear	,,	105
Raspberry Fool	,,	138
Raspberry Ripple Mousse	,,	122
Strawberry Fool	,,	133
Strawberry Mousse	,,	104
Strawberry Secret	,,	137
Strawberry & Vanilla Mousse	1 individual	110

Ice cream

Ice cream made with milk can be fairly nourishing although in all types of ice cream there is a fairly high carbohydrate content. Nevertheless, as long as it is eaten as part of a main meal and not as an extra snack, ice cream can help to add variety to a slimming diet and is not a particularly high calorie dessert. As with drinks, sweets, crisps and so on, ice cream can easily be left out of your calculations when you have it in between meals so that your total calorie consumption may be quite a bit higher than you think. It is this aspect which anyone with the slightest tendency to overweight needs to watch most carefully.

Food	Quantities	Calories
ICE CREAM		
Lyons		
Cornish Bar	1 bar	122
Cornish Mivvi	,,	86
Family Brick—		
vanilla	Whole brick	474
flavours	,, ,,	465
Glory Kup	1 portion	100
Handy Pack		
vanilla	1 portion	312
flavours	,, ,,	300
Vanilla Bar		
standard	1 bar	64
large	,,	99

Food	Quantities	Calories
Ross Frozen Foods		
Dairy Vanilla Ice Cream	2 oz portion	68
Standard Vanilla Ice Cream	2 oz portion	64
Rowntree's Ice Cream Powder	2 oz portion made up as directed with water	90
St. Ivel Readymix Ice Cream Powder	2 oz portion made up	102
Walls		
Non Milk Fat Ice Cream		
Coconut Nice	1 portion	148
Cornet Pieces	,, ,,	56
Dark & Golden Choc Bar	,,	130
Funny Faces	,,	62
Golden Vanilla Choc Bar	,,	128
Hazelnut Royal	,,	171
Midnight Mint	,,	137
Pink Elephant	,,	112
Standard Brickette	,,	77
Tubs	1 tub	90
Family Sweets—		
Strawberry	1 litre pack	931
Vanilla	,, ,,	956
Chocolate Ripple	One 483 ml. pack	531
Raspberry Ripple	,, ,, ,,	523
Strawberry Ripple	,, ,, ,,	520
Italian Style	,, ,, ,,	515
Orange Crush	,, ,, ,,	521
Dairy Ice Cream		
Cornish Brickettes	One brickette	80
Cornish Tub	One tub	98

Food	Quantities	Calories
Family Sweets—		
Rich Chocolate	One 483 ml. pack	573
Cornish	One litre pack	904
Cornish Raspberry		
Ripple	One litre pack	997
Cornish Dairy	One 483 ml. pack	431
Rich Strawberry	,, ,, ,,	487
Rich Vanilla	,, ,, ,,	521
Water Ices		
Orange Woppa & others		
average	One portion	30
Cinema Lines		
Choc'n Nut Cup	One portion	168
Cornish & Strawberry Cup	,, ,,	150
Dark & Cornish Choc Bar	,, ,,	131
Orange/Pineapple Split	,, ,,	77
Peach Parfait	,, ,,	122
Raspberry Velva Choc Bar	,, ,,	163
Rich Vanilla Cup	,, ,,	139

Biscuits

Biscuits are a quickly eaten, relatively concentrated form of energy food. Because they are crisp and crunchy and not very bulky it's easy to eat a lot of them. If you have a weight problem, check the calories carefully and if you are on a low calorie slimming diet you might be wise to choose bulkier, low calorie foods for as long as you are on the diet.

Food	Quantities	Calories
SAVOURY BISCUITS		
Crawford's		
Cream Crackers	1 biscuit	38
Tuc	,, ,,	26
Jacob's		
Biscuits for Cheese	,, ,,	15–35
Cream Cracker	,, ,,	36
Water Biscuits	,, ,,	35
Paterson's Farmhouse		
Oatcakes	1 biscuit	96
Rakusen's		
Crisp Crackers	1 biscuit	18
Small Table Crackers	,, ,,	15
Superfine Matzo's	,, ,,	18
Tea Matzo's	,, ,,	15
Wheaten Crackers	,, ,,	20
SWEET BISCUITS		
B.N. Biscuits		
Boudoir	1 biscuit	20
Macaroon	,, ,,	23

Food	Quantities	Calories
Cadbury's Chocolate Biscuits	Average per oz— fully covered biscuits highest	145–160
Carr's		
Milk Chocolate Lunch	1 biscuit	123
Plain Chocolate Lunch	,, ,,	122
Milk Chocolate Sports	,, ,,	113
Plain Chocolate Sports	,, ,,	113
Crawford's		
Butter Puffs	1 biscuit	50
Chocolate Wholemeal	,, ,,	78
Creamy Chocolate	,, ,,	71
Custard Creams	,, ,,	72
Ginger Snap	,, ,,	33
Glengarry	,, ,,	50
Marie	,, ,,	32
Rich Tea	,, ,,	40
Shortbread	1 oz	150
Thin Arrowroot	1 biscuit	32
Energen Starch Reduced		
Digestive	1 biscuit	39
Jacob's		
Buttercrisp	1 biscuit	43
Chocolate Thins	,, ,,	42
Club Fruit	,, ,,	130
,, Milk	,, ,,	130
,, Orange	,, ,,	130
,, Plain	,, ,,	128
Milk Chocolate Mallows	,, ,,	52
Milk Chocolate Wholemeal	1 biscuit	76
Plain Chocolate Wholemeal	1 biscuit	76
Puff Cracknel	,, ,,	21

Food	Quantities	Calories
Zing	1 biscuit	110
Macdonald's		
Bandit	1 biscuit	103
Fruit Sundaes	,, ,,	92
Mint Yo Yo	,, ,,	100
Munchmallow	,, ,,	80
Penguin	,, ,,	140
Taxi	,, ,,	87
Macfarlane Lang		
Abbey Crunch	1 biscuit	47
Butter Osborne	,, ,,	35
Fruit Shortcake	,, ,,	48
Granola	,, ,,	57
Princess	,, ,,	50
Rich Abernethy	,, ,,	59
Vienna Wafer	,, ,,	50
Mackie's		
Castle Shortbread Finger	1 biscuit	95
Petticoat Tail Shortbread	,, ,,	85
McVitie & Price		
Alibi	1 biscuit	116
Butter Crumble	,, ,,	40
Chocolate Digestive	,, ,,	130
Chocolate Homewheat	,, ,,	85
Chumbles	,, ,,	74
Digestive	,, ,,	70
Digestive Creams	,, ,,	74
Ginger Nuts	,, ,,	54
Gipsy Creams	,, ,,	82
Jaffa Cakes	,, ,,	50
Lincoln	,, ,,	45
Rich Marie	,, ,,	33
Rich Tea	,, ,,	35
Rondello	,, ,,	97

Food	Quantities	Calories
Royal Scot	1 biscuit	54
Shortcake	,, ,,	62
Snibs	,, ,,	49
Table Fingers	,, ,,	27
Thin Arrowroot	,, ,,	35
Wafer Fingers	,, ,,	47
Paterson's		
Highland Pack Shortbread	1 biscuit	87
Petticoat Tail Fingers	,, ,,	34
Rowntree's		
Breakaway Chocolate		
Digestive	1 oz	148
Kit Kat Chocolate Wafer	1 oz	146
Symbol		
Coconut Crunch Cake	1 biscuit	49
Ginger Crunch Cake	,, ,,	49
Maryland Cookie	,, ,,	50

Cakes

Tea is a meal which anyone who is worried about overweight might be wise to cut out completely and to some extent this goes for cakes as well. Of course, they can make a sweet course at a main meal but taken as an extra snack with morning coffee, at tea time or before going to bed at night they add very considerably to the day's total consumption of calories. They do have some nutritional value but there is a high proportion of carbohydrate and on a limited diet you might have to cut down on something nutritionally more valuable in order to make room for your slice of cake.

Food	Quantities	Calories
CAKES		
Lyons		
Baby Chocolate Rolls		
Choc. sponge, vanilla filled	1 roll	120
White sponge, jam filled	,,	106
Cup Cakes—		
chocolate, lemon, orange	1 cake	146
Harvest Sultana Cake	2 oz slice	178
Soufflette Sponges		
French jam	2 oz slice	182
Jam	,, ,,	174
Lemon	,, ,,	208
Sponge sandwiches-various	,, ,,	180
Sponge Cake individual	1 cake	87
Swiss Rolls—		
Choc. sponge, vanilla filled	2 oz slice	224
Choc. flavoured filling	,, ,,	218

Food	Quantities	Calories
Jam filled	2 oz slice	172
Jam & vanilla filled	,, ,,	200
Sponge Cake Mix		
(made up)	1 oz uncooked mix.	102
Mary Baker Cake Mixes		
Butterflies	1 oz cooked	131
Fruit Cake	⅛ cake, cooked	117
Economy Sponge	,, ,, ,,	160
Economy Chocolate		
Sponge	⅛ cake, cooked	155
Sandwiches	One tenth cake,	
	cooked	189
Scone	1 scone	90
Teatimers	1 oz, cooked	140
Tops	One	63
Viota Mixes		
Economical Plain Sponge	⅛ cake, cooked, 2	
	eggs recipe, no jam	98
Economical Rock Cakes	1 cake (12 to packet)	95
Economical Small Cakes	1 cake (,, ,,)	
	without currants	56
Economical Splits	1 cake (12 to pack)	
	without filling	52
Carnival Mix	1 cake (16 to pack)	63
Jam Sandwich	⅛ cake, cooked	
	& filled	172
Madeira Cake	One twelfth of	
	cake, cooked	125
Tea Cakes	1 cake (20 to pack)	71
Vanilla Sandwich	⅛ cake, cooked	
	& filled	200

Diet Foods

These are foods specially prepared for the slimmer. Some of them, but not all, are lower in calories than the equivalent, ordinary, food but generally the main difference is that vitamins and minerals have been added to compensate for any deficiencies which might otherwise arise in a poorly selected reducing diet. The manufacturers provide an analysis of the nutritional elements and give advice on using their products either as part of a calorie-controlled diet or as a full replacement for main meals over a limited period. If you observe these instructions, diet foods can be a useful aid. But do remember that no food is "slimming" in itself and if you eat diet foods in addition to ordinary meals you will never lose weight.

Food	Quantities	Calories
DIET FOODS		
Allinson Starch reduced rolls		
see *Cereal Products: Breads and Crispbreads* section		
Bisks		
Barbecued Chicken	1 biscuit	51
Cheese and Celery	,,	50
Chocolate Cream	,,	57
Chocolate Wholemeal	,,	72
Coffee Cream	,,	58
Cream Crackers	,,	35
Custard Cream	,,	66
Milk Chocolate Biscuits	,,	133
Orange Cream	,,	58

Food	Quantities	Calories
Plain Chocolate Biscuits	1 biscuit	134
Savoury Beef	,,	54
Sweetmeal (Digestive)	,,	46
Vienna Wafer	,,	54
Water Biscuits	,,	27
Water Biscuits (Small)	,,	12
Peppermint Creams	1 cream	68
Muesli Bar	1 bar	167
Plain Chocolate Bar	,,	313
Milk Chocolate Bar	,,	310
Hazelnut Chocolate	,,	310
Orange Wafer	,,	370
Fruit and Nut Chocolate	,,	320
Chocolate Wafer Bars	,,	108
Chocolate Nut Cookie	,,	45

Energen rolls etc—see *Cereal Products: Breads and Crispbreads*

Granose rolls etc—see *Cereal Products: Breads and Crispbreads*

Limmits
Biscuits

Choc-Mint	1 biscuit	140
Coffee	,, ,,	140
Lemon and Lime	,, ,,	140
Orange	,, ,,	140
Vanilla	,, ,,	140

Crackers

Cheese	1 biscuit	74
Lemon	,, ,,	74

Food	Quantities	Calories
Chocolate Bars		
Fruit & Nut Chocolate	1 meal	290
Hazelnut Chocolate	,, ,,	300
Milk Chocolate	,, ,,	290
Orange Chocolate	,, ,,	450
Peppermint Chocolate	,, ,,	450
Plain Chocolate	,, ,,	330
Chocolate Shortcake	1 biscuit	65
Chocolate Waffles	,, ,,	71
Lemon Waffles	,, ,,	71
Milk Chocolate Wholemeal	1 biscuit	71
Plain Chocolate Wholemeal	1 biscuit	71
Plain Shortcake	,, ,,	65
Plain Sweetmeal Digestive	,, ,,	50
Savouries		
Barbecued Chicken	1 biscuit	44
Cheese & Onion	,, ,,	44
Smoky Bacon	,, ,,	44
Trimmets		
Biscuits		
Bourbon	1 biscuit	72
Lemon-Choc	,, ,,	72
Orange	,, ,,	72
Chocolate Fingers	,, ,,	39
Crunch Cakes	,, ,,	115
Lemon Crunch Creams	,, ,,	83
Lemon Crisps	,, ,,	44
Savouries		
Beefburger	1 biscuit	44
Cheese & Ham	,, ,,	44
Trimmers	,, ,,	40
Turkey Sandwich	,, ,,	50

Food	Quantities	Calories
Vanilla Crunch Creams	1 biscuit	83
Wafers		
Chocolate	1 biscuit	70
Orange	,, ,,	70
Vanilla	,, ,,	70

Spreads

While meat, fish and cheese spreads may have a fairly high nutritional content, according to their quality, most jams and sweet spreads are purely carbohydrate and therefore their chief value is as energy foods. Spreads are intended to be tasty and easy to eat and can easily lead to a large consumption of bread so slimmers should be wary and keep a check on what they consume.

Food	Quantities	Calories
SPREADS;		
Savoury Spreads		
Burgess		
Anchovy Paste	¼ oz (1 hpd. tspn.)	10
Sardine & Tomato	,, ,, ,,	10
Bovril	¼ oz (1 lvl. tspn.)	5
Cheese spreads—		
see *Dairy Foods: Cheese*		
Granose Peanut Butter	¼ oz (1 hpd. tspn.)	45
Heinz Sandwich Spread	,, ,, ,,	24
Marmite	At 2 calories per oz	negligible
Princes		
Beef Spread	¼ oz (1 hpd. tspn.)	8
Chicken Spread	,, ,, ,,	10
Crab Paté	,, ,, ,,	8
Ham Spread	,, ,, ,,	18
Lobster Paté	,, ,, ,,	7
Salmon Spread	,, ,, ,,	9
Salmon & Shrimp Spread	,, ,, ,,	8
Sardine & Tomato Spread	,, ,, ,,	15
Turkey Spread	,, ,, ,,	9

Food	Quantities			Calories
Shippams				
Minced Foods—				
Dressed Crab with Butter	¼ oz (1 hpd. tspn.)			19
Minced chicken in jelly	,,	,,	,,	12
Minced turkey in jelly	,,	,,	,,	12
Potted Beef with Butter	,,	,,	,,	20
Potted Salmon with Butter	,,	,,	,,	18
Potted Sardine with Tomato	,,	,,	,,	13
Pastes				
Anchovy	¼ oz (1 hpd. tspn.)			17
Beef	,,	,,	,,	16
Bloater	,,	,,	,,	16
Chicken	,,	,,	,,	20
Chicken & Ham	,,	,,	,,	22
Crab	,,	,,	,,	18
Duck	,,	,,	,,	21
Ham & Beef	,,	,,	,,	23
Ham & Tongue	,,	,,	,,	23
Liver & Bacon	,,	,,	,,	21
Lobster	,,	,,	,,	19
Pilchard & Tomato	,,	,,	,,	14
Salmon & Anchovy	,,	,,	,,	17
Salmon & Shrimp	,,	,,	,,	17
Sardine & Tomato	,,	,,	,,	15
Turkey & Tongue	,,	,,	,,	20
Veal & Ham	,,	,,	,,	20
Spreads				
Beef Spread	,,	,,	,,	17
Chicken Spread	,,	,,	,,	17
Crab Paté	,,	,,	,,	15
Ham Spread	,,	,,	,,	18
Salmon Spread	,,	,,	,,	14
Sardine Spread	,,	,,	,,	16

Food	Quantities	Calories
Smoked Salmon Spread	¼ oz (1 hpd. tspn.)	13
Tongue Spread	,, ,, ,,	16
Sun-Pat		
Crunchy Peanut Butter	¼ oz (1 hpd. tspn.)	47
Smooth Peanut Butter	,, ,, ,,	47
Sweet Spreads		
Cadbury's Chocolate Spread	½ oz (2 tspns.)	43
Chivers jams—average	,, ,,	37
Frank Cooper		
Oxford Marmalade	,, ,,	48
**Diabetic Marmalade	,, ,,	44
Energen Low Sugar		
Jam or Marmalade	½ oz (2 tspns.)	25
Hartley's jams—average	,, ,,	37
Moorhouse jams—average	,, ,,	37
Robertson's jams, jelly jams & marmalade—average	,, ,,	36
Robertson's Mincemeat	1 oz (1 tbspn.)	71
Spring's		
Blue Cap Lemon Cheese	½ oz (2 tspns.)	41
Gold Cap Lemon Cheese	,, ,,	47
Lincolnshire Mincemeat	1 oz (1 tbspn.)	76
Traditional Mincemeat with Brandy	1 oz (1 tbspn.)	84
Orange Marmalade	½ oz (2 tspns.)	37

**Diabetic products are sweetened with products which are more suitable than ordinary sugar for diabetics but are not necessarily lower in calories.*

Pickles, Sauces and Relishes

It is impossible to generalise about the nutritional value of these products in themselves. Some are very high in calorie content—e.g. salad creams and mayonnaise—others are low, but what these products do have in common is that they help to make food more interesting and give it an extra zest. If you are trying to lose weight or are worried about your figure it is sensible to cut down on anything· that encourages you to eat more and to choose low-calorie rather than high-calorie products.

Food	Quantities	Calories
PICKLES, SAUCES & RELISHES		
Burgess		
Concentrated Mint Sauce	1 oz (1½ tbspns.)	12
Creamed Horseradish	½ oz (2 tspns.)	52
Mushroom Ketchup	¼ oz (1 teaspoon)	3
Sauce Tartare ·	1 oz (1½ tbspns.)	96
Chef Sauce	,, ,,	28
,, Tomato Ketchup	,, ,,	31
Crosse & Blackwell		
Boston Pickle	1 oz (1½ tbspns.)	30
Branston Pickle	,, ,,	37
Branston Sauce	,, ,,	26
French Capers	,, ,,	negligible
Gherkins	,, ,,	,,
Milder Mustard Pickle	,, ,,	15
Mixed Pickle	,, ,,	negligible
Piccalilli	,, ,,	7

Food	Quantities	Calories
Pickled Onions:		
brown, white & cocktail	1 oz (1½ tbspns.)	negligible
Pickled Walnuts	,, ,,	10
Salad Cream	,, ,,	114
Stuffed Manzanilla Olives	,, (app. 5 olives)	14
Sweet Mixed Pickle	,, (1½ tbspns.)	37
Tomato Pickle	,, ,,	41
Vinegar, malt or distilled	,, ,,	negligible
Heinz		
Ideal Sauce	,, ,,	33
Mayonnaise	,, ,,	98
Tomato Ketchup	,, ,,	29
Salad Cream	,, ,,	122
HP		
Fruity Sauce	1 oz (1½ tbspns.)	22
Sauce	,, ,,	25
Tomato Ketchup	,, ,,	32
Kraft		
Barbecue Sauce	,, ,,	32
Tartare Sauce	,, ,,	74
Lea & Perrins		
Worcestershire Sauce	as used, at 20 calories per oz,	negligible
Pan-Yan		
Curry Pickle	1 oz (1½ tbspns.)	45
Mango Pickle	,, ,,	50
Standard	,, ,,	45
Sweet	,, ,,	50

Drinks

Nutritionally speaking the important drinks are those containing milk; the rest may have some value, according to their Vitamin C content, but otherwise they simply provide a pleasant flavour and more or less energy according to their sugar or alcohol content. Drinks, particularly those low in calories, can help to stave off hunger pangs if you are dieting. On the other hand, it is easy to forget that drinks *do* contain calories and may contribute to an overweight problem.

Food	Quantities	Calories
DRINKS		
Alcoholic		
For more details see		
Jane Colin's Pocket Calorie		
Guide.		
Beer—average	Half pint	80
Cider—average	,, ,,	110
Sherry—average	1 sherry glass	75
Spirits—70% proof	1 sm. measure (1oz)	63
Wines—average	1 wineglass (5 oz)	90
Fruit Juices, Squashes and		
Carbonated drinks		
Britvic Fruit juices		
Grapefruit	4 fl. oz bottle	70
Orange	,, ,,	70
Pineapple	,, ,,	65
Tomato	,, ,,	25
Tomato Juice Cocktail	,, ,,	25

Food	Quantities	Calories
Canada Dry		
Bitter Lemon	10 oz bottle	104
Ginger Ale	,, ,,	91
Shandy Bass	,, ,,	62
Tonic Water	,, ,,	65
Low-Calorie products	At under $1\frac{1}{2}$ calories per fl. oz	negligible
Findus Frozen Fruit Juices		
Grapefruit Juice	5 oz glass (diluted as direc.)	60
Orange Juice	,, ,, ,,	65
Heinz		
Grapefruit	$4\frac{1}{2}$ oz can	46
Orange	,, ,,	63
Pineapple	,, ,,	67
Tomato	,, ,,	19
Idris Ginger Beer	6 oz serving	81
Libby's		
Unsweetened Grapefruit Juice	4 oz serving	44
Sweetened Grapefruit Juice	,, ,,	60
Unsweetened Orange Juice	,, ,,	52
Sweetened Orange Juice	,, ,,	60
Tomato Juice	,, ,,	20
Lucozade	6 oz serving	125
Pepsi-Cola	,, ,,	76
PLJ Lemon	1 oz ($1\frac{1}{2}$ tbspns.)	4
Quosh		
Blackcurrant Flavour Cordial	1 oz ($1\frac{1}{2}$ tbspns.)	39
Lemon Barley	,, ,,	34
Lemon Drink	,, ,,	31
Lemon & Lime	,, ,,	28
Lime Flavour Cordial	,, ,,	26

Food	Quantities	Calories
Orange Drink	1 oz (1½ tbspns.)	32
Orange & Pineapple Drink	,, ,,	28
Pineapple & Grapefruit Drink	1 oz (1½ tbspns.)	33
Raspberry Flavour Cordial	,, ,,	36
Tropical Fruit Drink	,, ,,	34
Peppermint Flavour Cordial	,, ,,	34
Ribena	,, ,,	84
Robinson's		
Whole Fruit Drink		
Grapefruit	1 oz (1½ tbspns.)	27
Lemon	,, ,,	27
Orange	,, ,,	31
Lemon Barley Water	,, ,,	30
Rose's Lime Juice Cordial	,, ,,	29
Schweppes		
Carbonated Drinks		
American Dry Ginger Ale	6 oz serving	60
Bitter Lemon Drink	,, ,,	52
Caribbean Lemon	,, ,,	55
Dry Ginger Ale	,, ,,	23
Ginger Beer	,, ,,	63
Lemonade	,, ,,	52
Sparkling Orange	,, ,,	78
Lemonade Shandy	,, ,,	50
Tonic Water	,, ,,	56
Cresta		
Lemon/Lime flavour	6 oz serving	95
Orange flavour	,, ,,	103
Pineapple flavour	,, ,,	103
Strawberry flavour	,, ,,	103
Slimline		
American Dry Ginger Ale	6 oz serving	negligible

Food	Quantities	Calories
Bitter Lemon Drink	6 oz serving	negligible
Sparkling Golden Orange	,, ,,	,,
Tonic Water	,, ,,	,,
Zing		
Lemonade	6 oz serving	68
Lemon/Lime	,, ,,	69
Orange	,, ,,	78
Raspberryade	,, ,,	75
Shloer		
Apple Juice	6 oz serving	60
Grape Juice Drink	,, ,,	84
Suncrush Fruit Drinks		
Grapefruit	1 oz (1½ tbspns.)	34
Lemon	,, ,,	34
Lemon Barley	,, ,,	33
Lemon/Lime	,, ,,	25
Orange	,, ,,	33
Tangerine	,, ,,	33
John West Fruit Juices		
Grapefruit	¼ of 11 oz can	52
Orange	,, , ,,	52
Pineapple (unsweetened)	,, ,, ,,	71
Milk Drinks		
Cadbury's		
Bournville Cocoa	½ oz (1 hpd. tspn.)	66
	½ oz mixed with	
	6 ozs milk	180
Bournvita	1 oz (1 lvl. tbspn.)	112
—	1 oz mixed with	
	6 ozs milk	226
Red Label Drinking	1 oz (1 lvl. tbspn.)	112
Chocolate	1 oz mixed with	
	6 ozs milk	226

Food	Quantities	Calories
Horlicks Malted Milk	1 oz (1 lvl. tbspn.)	115
	1 oz mixed with 6 ozs milk	229
Ovaltine	Mixed as recomm. with 6 ozs milk	165
Ovaltine Drinking Chocolate	Mixed as recomm. with 6 ozs milk	180
Rowntree's Cocoa	½ oz (1 hpd. tspn.)	51
	½ oz mixed with 6 ozs milk	165